Step by Step

Wound Healing

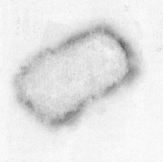

Step by Step
Wound Healing

Sylvie Meaume
Head Gerontologic Unit
Assistance Publique Hôpitaux de Paris
Hôpital Charles Foix
7, Avenue de la République
94205 Ivry/Seine France
0033149594507, Fax 00149594524
e-mail: sylvie.meaume@cfx.ap-hop-paris.fr
Expert in Management of Chronic Wounds
Director of the Wounds and Healings University Diploma Paris VI
Vice-President of the French Wound Healing Society
EPUAP Trustee
EWMA Editorial Board

Luc Téot
Burns and Plastic Unit
Hôpital Lapeyronie
391, Avenue du Doyen Gaston Giraud
34295 Montpellier Cedex
0033467338231, Fax 0033467041063
e-mail: l-teot@chu-montpellier.fr
Expert in management of acute and chronic wounds
Co-Director of the Wounds and Healings University Diploma
Montpellier I
President of the French Wound Healing Society
President Elect of the European Tissue Repair Society
President Elect of the World Union of Wound Healing Societies

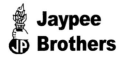

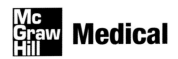

© 2005 Sylvie Meaume, Luc Téot

First published in India in 2004 by
  Jaypee Brothers Medical Publishers (P) Ltd, New Delhi, India
  EMCA House, 23/23B Ansari Road, Daryaganj, New Delhi 110 002, India
  Phones: 23272143, 23272703, 23282021, 23245672, Fax: +91-011-23276490
  e-mail: jaypee@jaypeebrothers.com, Visit our website: www.jaypeebrothers.com

First published in USA by The McGraw-Hill Companies, 2 Penn Plaza, New York, NY 10121.
Exclusively worldwide distributor except South Asia (India, Nepal, Sri Lanka, Bhutan, Pakistan, Bangladesh).

ISBN 0-07-145775-5

Preface

Wound healing has been the subject of a fantastic development since the last decade. The World Union of Wound Healing Societies represents a group of more than 5000 professionals spread all over the world, all members of the national groups and societies involved in wound healing. Techniques and management guidelines are still the subject of discussions in many continents, but it has been evidence based medicine demonstrated that the first mandatory step in wound management is the wound debridement. Debridement can be done by many different techniques, some of them being more progressive than others. The choice of the technique depends on the type of wound, the etiology, the degree of infection and the level of resources available. In this direction you can either choose a rapid expensive solution or a more progressive and safe cheap one.

Step by step debridement in wound healing represents the first issue of a long WUWHS Educational Program series.

Sylvie Meaume
Luc Téot

Acknowledgements

Our thanks and sincere gratitude to Christine Khavas from the Polyclinique and nurses from pavillon l'Orbe, in Clinics of Gerontology in Charles Foix Hospital, Thanks to Mrs Sylvie Palmier, Chloé Trial and Evelyne Ribal from Montpellier University Hospital.

Contents

Chapter 1

Definition: Rationales for Debridement

DEFINITION

Debridement is defined as "the removal of foreign material and dead or damaged tissue especially in a wound" in the *Taber's Cyclopedic Medical Dictionary*. It is well demonstrated that wound healing cannot take place if necrotic tissue is not removed. Devitalized tissue is a perfect medium for infection. Debridement is needed in all types of wounds, acute and chronic, whatever be the origin of the presence of necrotic, fibrous or sloughy tissues. Necrotic tissue is submitted to bacterial proliferation, inhibits phagocytosis and epithelial cell migration, prevents an accurate assessment of the wound bed, decreases antiseptics efficacy. Debridement reduces the number of germs and toxins in the wound bed.

Chapter 2

Types of Debridements

Several techniques of debridement are available (**Figure 2.1**). Clinician practicing wound healing should select the most appropriate technique to the patient's condition. Regardless the technique selected, the need to assess and control pain should always be considered. Different techniques can be proposed. The choice of the technique depends on the speed of debridement required, how selective it has to be, how painful the wound is. The amount of exudate, the presence of infection and the cost are also important factors to integrate.

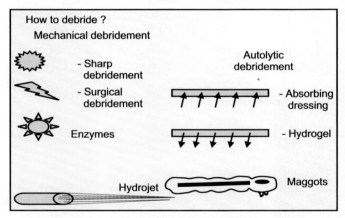

Figure 2.1: Different techniques of debridement

Mechanical Debridement

It includes surgical/sharp techniques, wet to dry techniques, use in dextranomers and pressure lavages (hydrojet) and negative pressure therapy.

Sharp/Surgical

Sharp/surgical is the fastest selective (little or no damage to the healthy tissue) technique, used alone or combined with others techniques.

- Surgical debridement was initially described by Chinese authors 5,000 years ago. This aggressive method can be done with surgical instruments, by a surgeon or a physician, usually in an operating room **(Figure 2.2)**. In the operating room, stop bleeding is more easy (electrocoagulation), pain prevention is done by specialists and a complete, wide "carcinologic" excision of the necrotic or doubtful tissues is possible.
- Sharp debridement is simple removal of thick, adherent eschar and devitalized tissues **(Figure 2.3)**

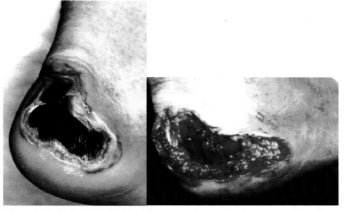

Figure 2.2: Surgical debridement shortens the wound healing, but there are few risks to adopt a more progressive attitude if no inflammation or infection is present

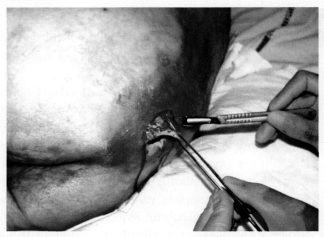

Figure 2.3: Sharp debridement using scalpel starts in the center of the necrotic process, then progresses circularly towards the peripheral zones

These technique is slightly less aggressive, and can be done with minimal instrumentation (scissors and scalpels) at the bedside, at home, in the clinician's office, by a physician or other licensed practitioner, trained healthcare professional, such as a nurse or a physical therapist or a podiatrist **(Figures 2.4 and 2.5)**.
- Using surgical tools outside the operating room has to respect two principles:
  1. No pain: Verbal prevention is realized by explaining to the patient is the next step and anticipate the possible sources of painful maneuvers. Non-traumatic techniques should be preferred, largely preparing the site by using local anesthesia. EMLA®

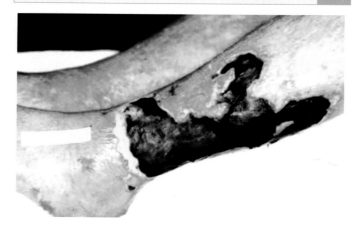

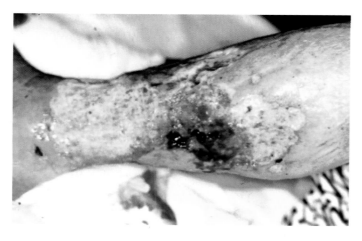

Figure 2.4: Debridement of a leg hematoma at the bedside of an elderly demented women in a geriatric wards

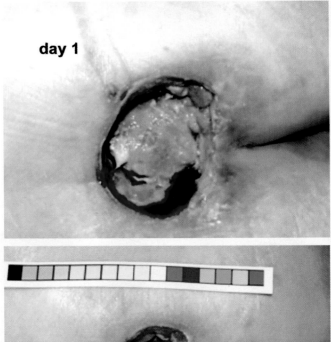

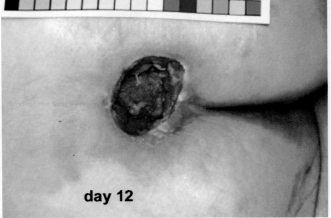

Figure 2.5: Sacral pressure sore at day 1 and day 12 after sharp debridement at bedside conducted by nurses during dressing change

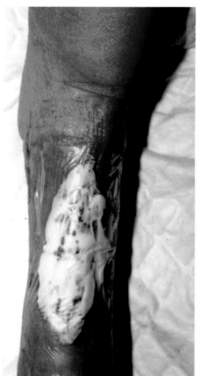

Figure 2.6: Pain is frequent and has to be prevent for example with EMLA® cream, applied at least 30 minutes before the debridement

cream can be used limited amount of times when applied directly on exposed dermis—8 times maximum. This cream is a mixture of two amide local anesthetics. The cream can be applied in a thick coat and covered with an adhesive film for 30 to 60 minutes before debridement **(Figure 2.6)**. Alternatively 1% to 4% xylocaine solution or gel has been topically used in some clinical settings.

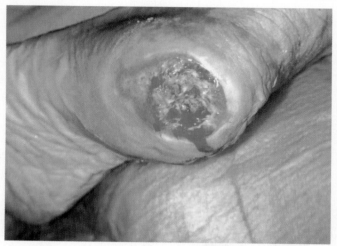

Figure 2.7: Debridement is successfull when obtaining a well bleeding wound, without any sloughy material, necrosed part or remaining fibrin

Otherwise, patient can be premedicated 30 to 60 minutes before debridement with oral analgesics (e.g. morphine).

2. No bleeding **(Figure 2.7)**: The extent of mechanical debridement must not overpass the edges of the healthy tissues, debriding progressively, partially and use complementary techniques: enzymes, hydrogels, cleansing, etc.

No stress must be shown by the practitioner during the technique of debridement which must be taught to each healthcare professional. Stress and fear to go too far are the main reasons of a poor management and the lack of equipments is often a false reason. Traps can be prevented by a good anticipation, a large experience and some tricks

- *Technical points:* Superficial curettage of adherent tissues can be done when necessary, in other situations a deep debridement is more prone to eliminate a large quantity of necrotic tissues (**Figures 2.8 and 2.9**). Traction should be exclusively applied on dead tissues, cutting parallel to the skin, without being afraid of enlarging the wound. Surgical debridement shortens

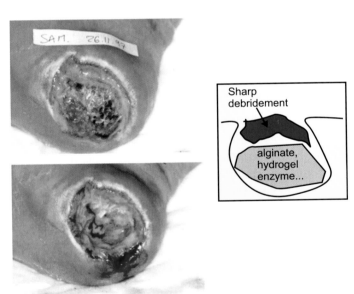

Figure 2.8: Sharp debridement of a heel pressure ulcer has to be completed by a progressive autolytic debridement using alginates

Debridement: A partnership

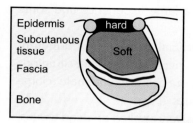

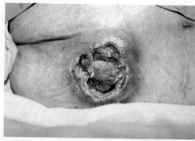

Figure 2.9: Debridement at the bedside can sometimes expose bone (in case of pressure ulcers stage IV)

drastically the healing process and the outcome is better in difficult situations where necrotic infected tissues interfere with limb salvage. Adapted instruments must be used (single use or sterilizable instruments). Reinforced dissection scissors, curve and straight should be preferred. Forceps with jaws can be applied only on dead tissues. Blade selection can be done by using blade 15 for perincision, 23 for hard tissues, 11 for incision or drainage.

Wet to Wet and Wet to Dry Techniques

In wet to dry, moistening one layer of wide-mesh cotton gauze with saline is usually achieved, wringing it out until it is just damp, applying it to the wound bed, allowing it to dry before removing.

In wet to wet, irrigation must be maintained for the whole period of time between two successive dressings, and it is not allowed to dry out before removal.

These techniques are non-selective, can remove viable tissue, remain traumatic for granulation tissue (**Figure 2.10**), a freshly formed epithelial tissue, are painful and require adequate analgesia, its present risks of bleeding at each dressing change (**Figure 2.11**).

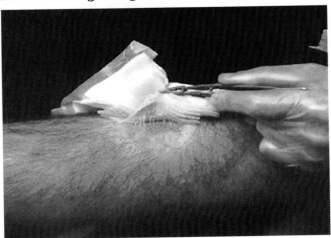

Figure 2.10: Wet to dry technique is non-selective, removes viable tissue and is traumatic for granulation tissue, and freshly epithelialised tissue

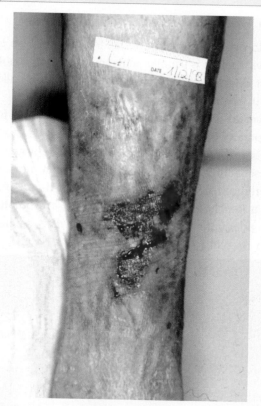

Figure 2.11: Wet to dry technique is painful, requires an adequate analgesia. Risks of bleeding are present

Osmotic Debridement

It can be done using Dextranomer (Debrisan®), or hypertonic saline (Mesalt®, Hypergel®).

This technique allow exudate absorption, get away germs and dead cells from the wound bed. Dressing should

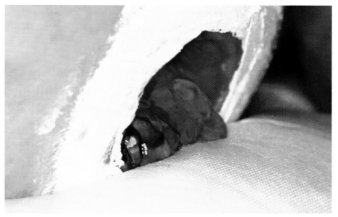

Figure 2.12: Osmotic debridement with Hypergel®. Protection of peri-wound is need to prevent irritation and pain with hypersaline gel

be changed daily. Osmotic debridement is difficult to apply, sometimes painful for a few hours after dressing change **(Figure 2.12)**.

Hydrojet Debridement and/or Pulsatile Pressure Cleansing

Depending on the level of pressure proposed, different types of materials are available: high pressure (Versajet®, Debritom®) or low pressure (Jetox®, Surgilav®). They are used as a helper to debridement. Some of them can be very expensive, not always safe due to the risks of spreading germs in the surrounding ambiance, and not available everywhere. Cleansing the wound everyday is still an option to be promoted, even without high pressure. These cleansing solutions are adopted in some countries.

Tap water can be used in some countries where tap water presents a limited amount of germs and can be drunk.

Surgilav®

Surgilav® create hydrodebridement with saline pulse into the wound bed to debride. It cleans wound bed more than it debrides adherent tissues (pressure under 15 PSI). It is a homebound disposal and it can be done at home as it is non-invasive and doesn't cause trauma at the wound bed (**Figures 2.13 to 2.15**). This technique is some time painful, specially in leg ulcer.

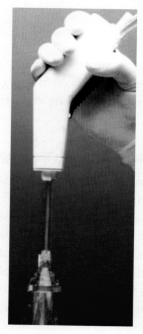

Figure 2.13: Surgilav® handpiece

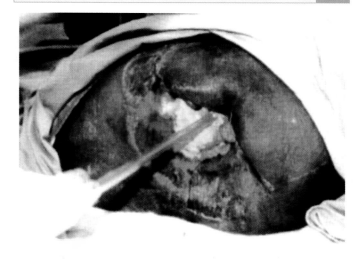

Figure 2.14: Debridement of pressure ulcer with Surgilav®

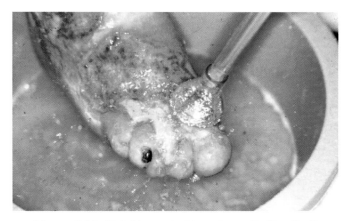

Figure 2.15: Debridement of leg ulcer with Surgilav®

Jetox®

Jetox® use compressed oxygen combined with saline solution. This modern technology use standard connectors for gas outlet and saline dispensers. It is available at the bedside and also at home for outpatients. Jetox® product family transform saline and oxygen into microdroplets and accelerate them to supersonic speed to form a powerful jet spray. The jet is precisely calibrated to treat only the affected skin area in the aim to debride gently and efficiently diabetic foot ulcers, pressure ulcers, venous leg ulcers, burn and difficult-to-heal tissue **(Figures 2.16 and 2.17)**.

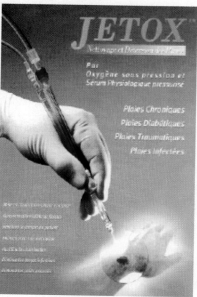

Figure 2.16: Jetox®

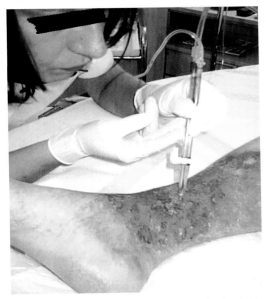

Figure 2.17: Nurse debride a leg ulcer at the bedside with Jetox®

Debritom®

This equipment is composed of a high pressure command unit, a metallic tube linked to the handpiece, and a pressure air bottle (Figure 2.18). The pump aspirates NaCl (0.9%), which is directed through the high pressure tube to the handpiece. The pressure can vary by adaptation of working distance or using a pressure regulation system (from 0 to 800 bars). This equipment can be transported easily in different sites. The liquid is ejected distal to the handpiece through a "buse". Cutting, dissecting and washing can be achieved on demand, and

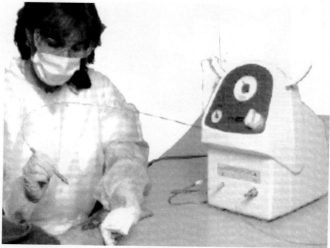

Figure 2.18: Debritom® is a high pressure debrider, necessitating some precautions in term of projections of contaminated materials

shifting from one to the other is very easy. So, this system can be used as a powerful bistoury if needed (**Figure 2.19**).

Clinical results show an important reduction of necrotic tissue and fibrin (**Figure 2.20**) and a better aspect of wounds in 2 interventions only (spaced from 2 to 3 days) (**Figure 2.21**). The medium pressure used was about 300 bar. Major problems of using these techniques are linked to the equipments themselves which needs good team teaching. Waste projection risk is important, so; infectious dissemination risk is probably important for the nurse as for the environment surfaces! Cost is important because of using disposable materials: handpieces, tubes,

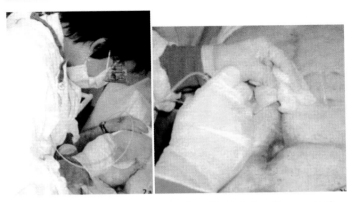

Figure 2.19: The pressure obtain with Debritom® can reach 400 bars through a finely manufactured endpiece

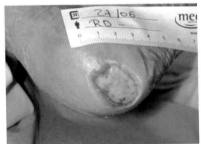

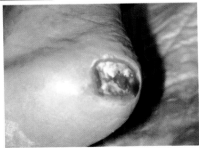

Figure 2.20: Heel pressure ulcer debride with Debritom®

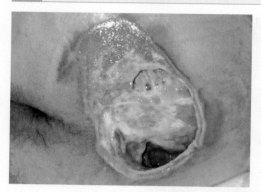

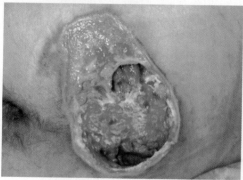

Figure 2.21: Sacral pressure ulcer
debride with Debritom®

etc. and Debritom® needs a disinfectant solution and sterile
wearing for the nurse which add time and money
difficulties. The Debritom® can be useful to treat cavity
wounds even if the access hole is small. If the wound is
full of black necrotic tissue, debridement has to be done

with classic scalpel (without pain) for the first time and waterjet will be useful in a second time.

Versajet®

The equipment is composed of a high pressure command unit which pressurizes the NaCl (without pressure air bottle), and a disposable handpiece. Waste water and the debridement products are sucked back inside the handpiece and driven to a waste container (less risk of projection). The maximal pressure is 827 bars. Pressure can only be adapted by the system of regulation, due to the configuration of the handpiece. Three different working angles are available as handpieces, allowing to adapt to the geometry of the different wounds. Because of this configuration, Versajet® cannot be compared to a scalpel but looks more like a curette (so, the cutting of black necrotic tissue is not possible and has to be realized or achieved previously). Versajet® was evaluated in Germany as an efficient tool, safe, without causing any damage to the surrounding tissues, and easy to handle by any practitioner. The usage of these new techniques shows that their interest is against fibrin even in important quantity. Little spottings appears since the first use, stimulating blood flow.

Negative Pressure Therapy (Vacuum Assisted Closure®)

Negative pressure therapy can be considered as a good tool to clean the wound after a gross debridement, when necrotic tissue has been removed and even if sloughy tissue is still present. NPT is a good absorbing device for exudates and is more effective in promoting the granulation tissue progression.

Efficacy of negative pressure therapy is reduced when a large undermined cavity is poorly drained by the aspirative foam dressing.

Negative pressure therapy is not indicated in presence of bone infection, of malignant wound and when necrotic tissue is persisting on the surface of the wound.

A short training is necessary before use. Even if the cost is high, this technique is cost-effective, even in emerging countries **(Figures 2.22 to 2.26)**

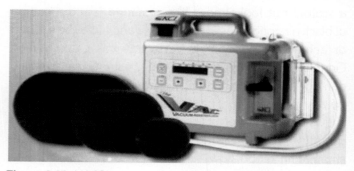

Figure 2.22: VAC® is a negative pressure from 25 to 200 mm Hg created by a pump, applied over the wound when exudates are important, in case of cavity wound, acute or chronic, after mechanical debridement. It includes tube and connections, a polyurethane foam and adhesive PU films to create vacuum

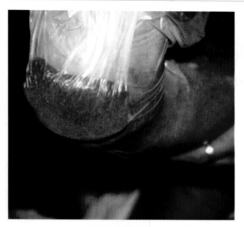

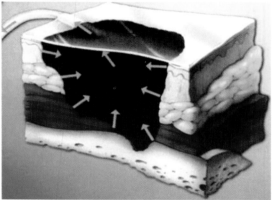

Figure 2.23: Negative pressure therapy is indicated at the end of debridement in trauma wounds after parage, in chronic wounds when there is no more necrotic tissue, in paraplegic patients. Local soft tissue infection is not a contraindication. On the contrary, osteitis and cancer wounds are a contraindication for VAC

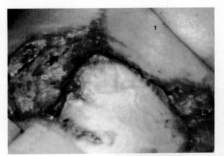

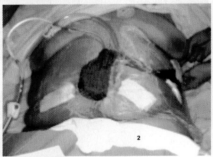

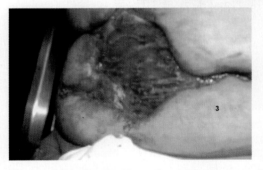

Figure 2.24: Eventration after intestine resection for a Crohn disease. Failure of a rotation flap. VAC® for 21 days: (1) abdominal wall tissue loss to debride, (2) VAC® in place, (3) after 21 days, wound ready to graft

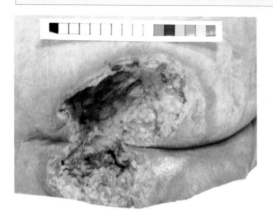

Day 0

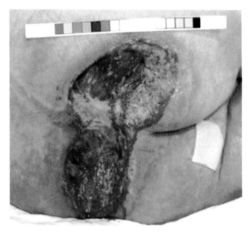

Day 25

Figure 2.25: VAC® In spite of a rapid progression of the granulation tissue, muscular areas are more reluctant to granulate when devascularization has been extensive and long. Discrepancies in healing speed are often observed in different areas of the same wound

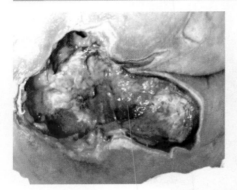

Day 0

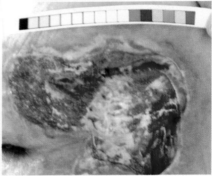

Day 20

Figure 2.26: VAC® Clinical evolution is some time tricky: in this case, most of the sacral pressure ulcer has been changed from necrotic tissue to granulation tissue. However, a laterally located undermined area will prevent a good evolution. Infection can develop in this area

Enzymatic Debridement

Enzymatic debridement is slower and less aggressive than sharp debridement. This method is a good alternative for non-infected, non-complicated wounds. Dressing has to be changed at least once a day (preferably 2 or 3 times a day). Gauze is used as secondary dressing. Different products are launched

- Krill enzymes coming from digestive secretions of krills
- Collagenase (Iruxol®, Santyl®)
- Fibrinolysin and deoxyribonuclease ± chloromycetin (Elase®)
- Papain (Panafyl®) ± urea (Gladase®, Accuzyme®)
- Debridase, high concentrations of bromelaine

Some transient sensation of "burning" can be observed immediately after application. Evidence Based Medicine proofs are weak on all these products but they are widely used. Cutting or cross-hatching using a scalpel through the depth of black necrosis allows the enzymatic agent to penetrate faster inside the wound.

Biological Debridement (Maggots)

One type of maggot has been proposed by several authors (Lucila Sericata, which does not harm the wound bed), presented as isolated maggots **(Figures 2.27 and 2.28)** or a group included in a biobag. This technique, which is a common practice since 1930s has begun to be widely spread all over the world and has been credited to provoke a rapid selective debridement. Some countries have adviced the use of maggots as the first choice technique when debriding diabetic foot ulcer.

Larvae secrete highly proteolytic enzyme (collagenase which hydrolyzes denatured protein), calcium salts and antimicrobial agents. Maggots create some mechanical irritation due to the movement of chewing and reducing bacterial counts. Maggots promote wound healing, stimulate the production of a serous exudate, reduce the bacterial concentration, promote the granulation tissue formation. The clinical indications are local chronic infection, osteitis, burns and acute infections. Biological debridement is indicated for narrow, deep, with irregular edge wounds instead of sharp debridement. The selectivity in debridement obtained with these living organisms is superior to others, their feeding being preferentially done by liquefying necrotic tissues and devascularized areas.

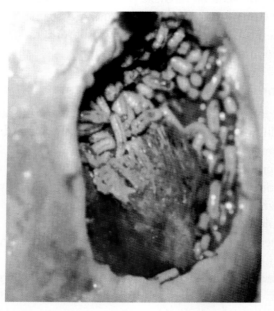

Figure 2.27: Biological debridement by fly larvae (maggots)

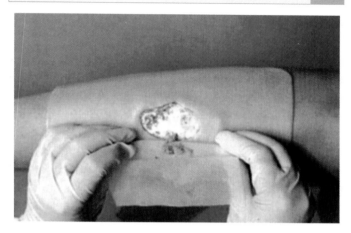

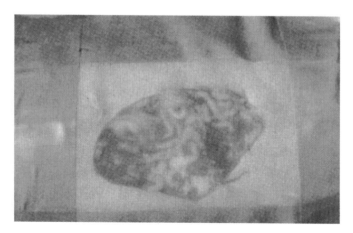

Figure 2.28: The maggots dressing includes protection of the peri-wound with hydrocolloid, transfer of the larvae on the wound bed and cover with a secondary dressing

Autolytic Debridement

The principle is to use the body's own digestive enzyme to break down necrotic tissue (**Figure 2.29**). Autolysis is accomplished by maintaining the wound moist with retentive dressing occlusive: hydrocolloids (**Figures 2.30 to 2.34**), foams (**Figures 2.35 and 2.36**), or non-occlusive: alginate (**Figures 2.37 to 2.40**), hydrofiber (**Figures 2.41 to 2.43**) and hydrogels (**Figures 2.44 and 2.45**). Autolytic debridement is a selective method, painless, slower than surgical debridement. This method can be used alternatively or complementary to mechanical debridement. Dressings used can be classical impregnated gauze or ointments (Mebo®) or advance wound care dressings like alginates, hydrofiber, hydrocolloids or foams.

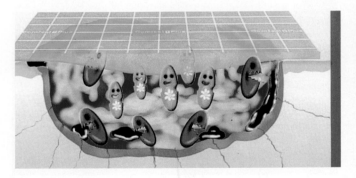

Figure 2.29: Autolytic debridement is a slow process of elimination of necrotic tissues absorbed in the dressing, combined with the moist environment brought by the dressing, which helps to bring humidity to the remaining hard necrotic parts

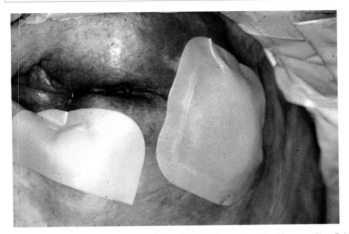

Figure 2.30: Hydrocolloids (HC)(*Comfeel®, Granuflex®/ Duoderm®, Hydrocoll®, Tegasorb®*) *are* the most widely used modern dressing. These dressing contains gel-forming agent (Na-CMC, gelatin) combined with elastomer and adhesives applied to a carrier (polyurethane foam or film)

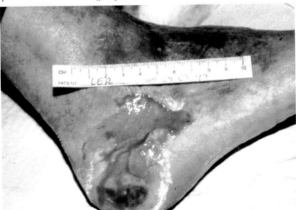

Figure 2.31: In presence of exudate, hydrocolloids absorbs liquid and forms a malodorous gel

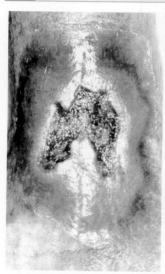

Figure 2.32: Hydrocolloid is recommended for low to mode-rate exudating wounds, for clean, granulating, superficial wounds, when the surrounding skin is intact

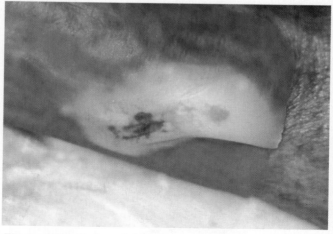

Figure 2.33: Hydrocolloid dressings requires changing only every 3-7 days. Cost-effectiveness is therefore evidenced

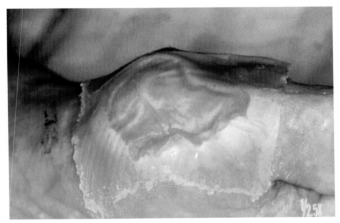

Figure 2.34: Hydrocolloid dressings provide an effective occlusion and a barrier against germs (prevent the MRSA spread)

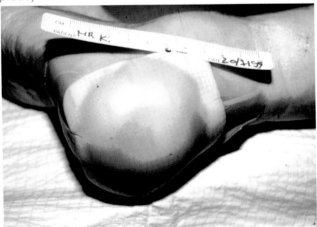

Figure 2.35: Foam dressing (*Allevyn®, Biatain®, Tielle® ...*) is promoted as an alternative to hydrocolloids. Significant differences were noted in favour of foams concerning a less dressing leakage and less odor production

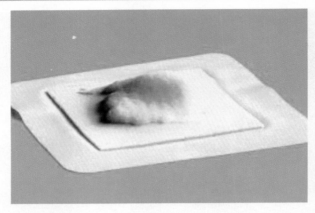

Figure 2.36: Foam dressing absorb more without leakage and produce less malodour

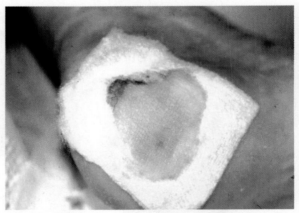

Figure 2.37: Alginate dressings (*Kaltostat®, Algisite®, Algosteril®, Seasorbsoft®, Melgisorb®, Sorbsan®, Urgosorb®* ...) are derived from seaweed. They are formed with a mixture of manuronic and guluronic acid ± carboxy-methyl-cellulosis. These dressings present high absorption capacities via a strong hydrophilic gel formation

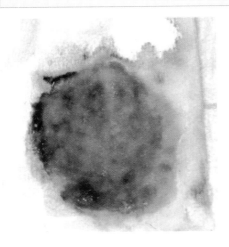

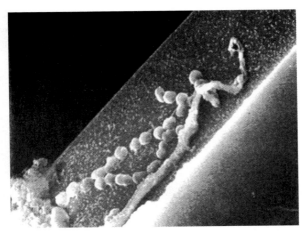

Figure 2.38: Alginate dressings help to prevent infection. At each dressing change bacteria which are adherent to alginate fibers are removed with the dressing. A green color of the dressing, due to *Pseudomonas aeruginosa*, is often observed

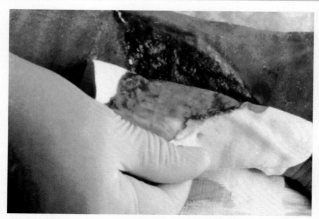

Figure 2.39: Alginate dressing can be soaked using saline solution irrigation. So, removal during dressing doesn't harm the granulation tissue. The dressing change is painless

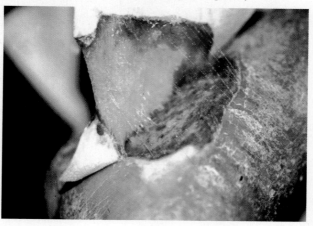

Figure 2.40: Alginate is indicated for moderate to heavily exudating wounds. Moisture can help to debride in addition with mechanical debridement

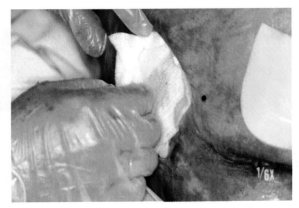

Figure 2.41: Aquacel® is an hydrofiber dressing made of textured carboxymethylcellulose which has the same indications than alginate dressing except the fact it is not hemostatic

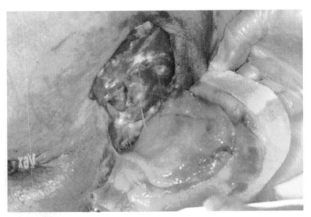

Figure 2.42: The proposed secondary dressing covering Aquacel is usually a hydrocolloid. A moist environment is so created under this occlusive dressing

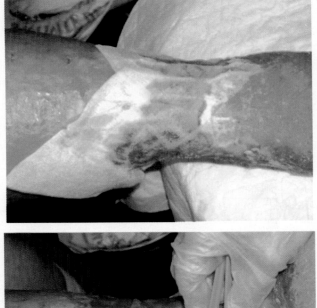

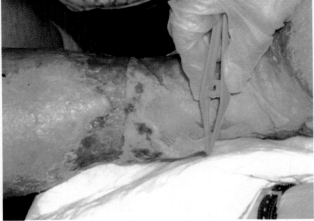

Figure 2.43: Autolytic debridement of venous leg ulcer with Aquacel® is a more progressive attitude if no inflammation or infection is present. Colonisation with *Pseudomonas aeruginosa* is not a contraindication

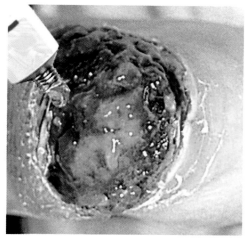

Figure 2.44: Hydrogel (*Intrasite ®, Purilon ®, Nu-gel ® ...*) is useful for dry, sloughy or necrotic wounds

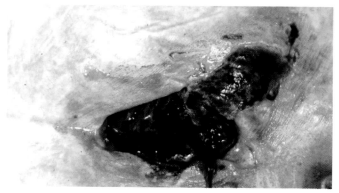

Figure 2.45: With hydrogel, appropriate secondary dressing is required (not absorbing). Hydrogels transform dry necrotic tissue into a moist necrotic one, easier to remove

Chapter 3

When to Debride and When not to Debride

DEBRIDE

Debridement should be proposed in case of deep eschar (Figures 3.1 and 3.2), purulence (Figures 3.3 and 3.4), infection (Figure 3.5), large area of necrosis (Figures 3.6 to 3.8). The choice of the techniques depends essentially on the training level of the practitioners, the amount of resources and the local disponibility of an operating room. Debridement should be done gradually when there is no infection (Figure 3.9), more aggressively in an infected area (Figure 3.10). Emergencies in debridement are deep trauma wounds, burns (Figure 3.11) and purpura fulminans necrotic zones discharging purulent materials in the blood vessels (Figure 3.12).

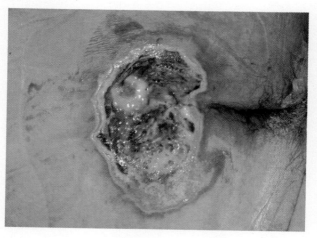

Figure 3.1: Yellow and black moist tissue has to be debrided in order to prepare wound healing

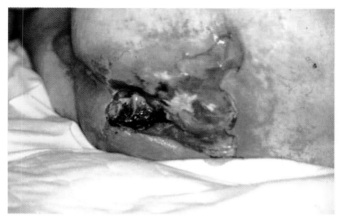

Figure 3.2: Sharp debridement of the dark tissue should be proposed. For the yellow one use autolytic debridement

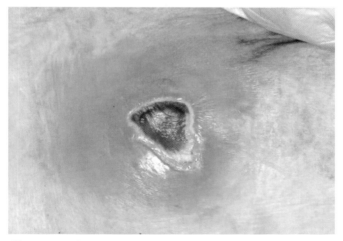

Figure 3.3: Debridement is mandatory when an abscess is collected

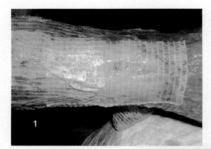

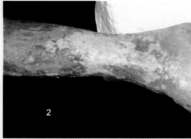

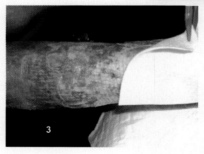

Figure 3.4: Infection due to *Pseudomonas aeruginosa* should rarely be submitted to any debridement. This infection does not harm seriously the wound healing process. Autolytic debridement is often enough. (1) leg ulcer with impregnated gauze, (2) leg ulcer with sloughy tissue to debride, (3) autolytic debridement with alginate dressing

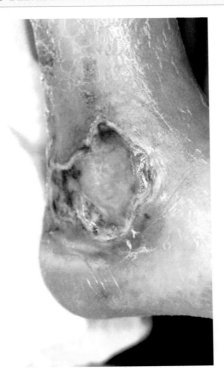

Figure 3.5: To prevent infection in this colonized leg ulcer with *Pseudomonas aeruginosa* (green color) a simple foot bath with tap water can be used (antiseptic are not required) to debride devitalized tissues

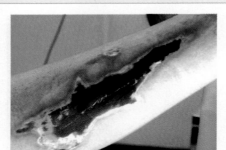

Figure 3.6: Necrosis of the posterior aspect of the leg in a 22 years old medical student who underwent a venous sclerosis using Thrombovar. The product was extravasated from the vein and provoked an extensive deep necrosis

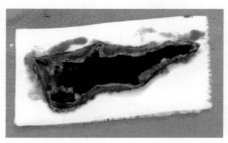

Figure 3.7: After surgical debridement, the necrosed tissue extends to 2 cm lateral to the apparent edges

Figure 3.8: When looking at the deep aspect of the debrided necrosis, one can see that the subcutaneous tissue is touched by the necrotic process

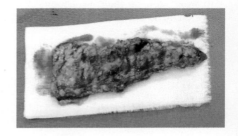

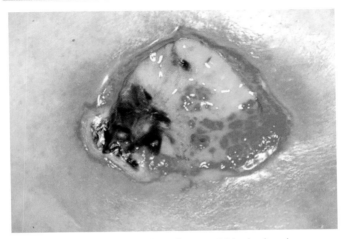

Figure 3.9: Debride yellow and black sloughy
moist and hard dry tissue

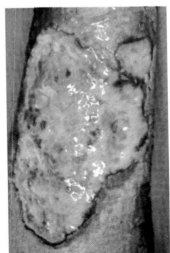

Figure 3.10: Debridement
should be done for this yellow
sloughy moist venous leg ulcer.
Association of an absorbent
dressing and a compression
bandaging will promote healing

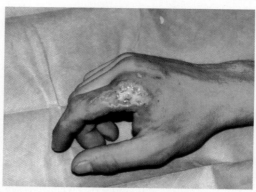

Figure 3.11: Electrical burns of the metacarpal area. The extent of necrotic tissue is better evaluated after some days. In this case, the risk of exposure of extensor tendons and the joint capsule are important. Coverage technique must be decided before debridement

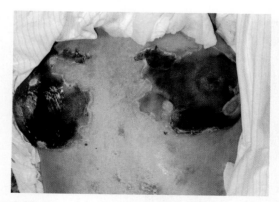

Figure 3.12: Necrotizing fasciitis is often observed after exposure to meningococcemia or streptococci group D. The necrotic process is extensive, brutal and deep. Debridement should not be realized early, before having evaluated all the amount of involved tissues

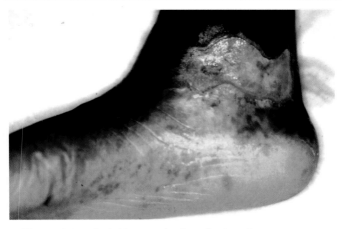

Figure 3.13: Debridement is done in the aim to promote granulation tissue formation in this non-granulating wound

Social considerations in end of life of HIV patients presenting large amounts of necrosis of nodes zones (axilla, groin) can create the need for a mild debridement for reduction of odor preventing the family to accompany the patient. Debridement sometimes promote granulation in a non-progressing wound, difficult to heal **(Figure 3.13)**

NOT DEBRIDE

Debridement should not be done when the wound is clean **(Figure 3.14)**, non-infected **(Figure 3.15)**, free of necrotic tissue, foreign matter or fibrin, when there is no tender fluctuation, erythema, suppuration. A heel pressure ulcer presenting a dry eschar **(Figure 3.16)** can be treated

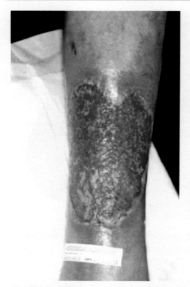

Figure 3.14: A small amount of yellow tissue is covering the wound bed of this venous leg ulcer: compression bandaging and autolytic debridement with dressing is enough to obtain epithelialization

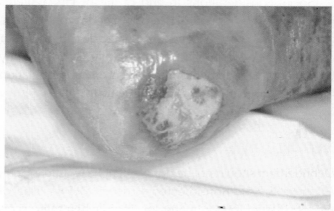

Figure 3.15: It is not absolutely needed to debride a non-infected wound, with few necrotic tissue, foreign matter or fibrin slough

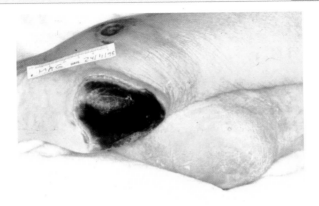

Figure 3.16: Heel pressure ulcer associated with arterial insufficiency with dry eschar need not to be debrided if edema, erythema, fluctuance or drainage are absent. This eschar provides a natural protective cover

without debridement if there is no drainage, fluctuance, pain or erythema. This eschar provides a natural protection until the edges begin to open. Dry gangrene or stable ischemic wound should not be amputated or debrided until the patient's vascular status can be improved by an adapted revascularization (Figures 3.17 and 3.18).

Superficial dermatologic lesions like Lyell syndromes and epidermolysis bullosa should not be debrided and left to specialists.

It is necessary to remind that one should wait before debriding when the difference between dead and still living tissues is not evident clinically (Figures 3.19 and 3.20). In malignant wounds, palliative care objective is not

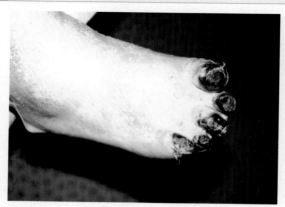

Figure 3.17: Dry gangrene or stable ischemic wound should be left in situ until the patient's vascular status can be improved in diabetic patient or elderly

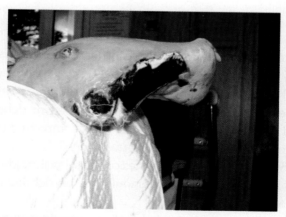

Figure 3.18: When the necrotic territory is completely determined, the discussion should be to amputate or not to amputate: In this dilemma, a good evaluation of the arterial supply should include an arteriogram, prior any decision from the vascular surgeon

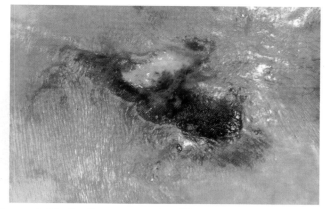

Figure 3.19: For the moment the difference between living and dead tissues is not clear, it is better to wait before debridement

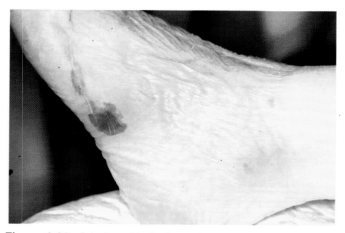

Figure 3.20: Arteriopathic lesions should not be debrided too early, especially when the ischemic process has not completely determined the necrotic territory

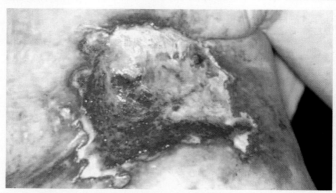

Figure 3.21: This patient has a breast cancer with no possibility of curative treatment. Palliative care is needed. Comfort and pain control are the main objectives. Try to debride smoothly to prevent infection, using autolytic debridement

to heal but to prevent complications or discomfort due to the wound **(Figure 3.21)**. In these situations the debridement will be less active.

Chapter 4

Types of Wound Shape

Wounds are not the same and, apart from etiologies, anatomical localization and speed of progression of necrotic tissue determine different types of wounds:

FLAT WOUNDS

Flat wounds (**Figure 4.1**) are sometime very extensive in term of surfaces. Burns, trauma wounds and leg ulcers provide large surfaces uncovered with skin. On these surfaces, wound healing potential is linked to the nature of the pathology.

• In burns, specifically in thermal burns, a toxin can be delivered by the local necrotic tissue accumulated over

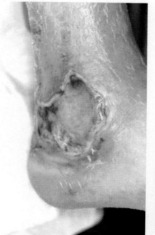
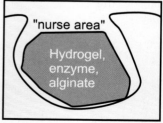

"nurse area"

Hydrogel, enzyme, alginate

Figure 4.1: Debridement must be understood as a partnership between professionals. An international "nurse area" has been defined by a consensus of wound healers

a 3rd degree burns. The devitalized area should be ideally rapidly excised and grafted by specialists.

- In trauma wounds degloving skin or provoking abrasions, the problem is the depth of the lesion and in some cases can be compared to burns.
- In leg ulcers, the wound sole is deeply recomposed by fibrin and non-healing surfaces, more or less infected. This type of wound has to be selectively cureted regularly, after local application of creams preventing pain during the debriding maneuver.

CAVITY WOUNDS

Cavity wounds are frequently observed during evolution of a pressure ulcer. Different cavities can be seen, depending on the local anatomical situation. In sacral PU, undermining due to the permanence of shearing forces is the cause of enlargement of the wound (Figures 4.2 and 4.3). Usually, these wounds have a tendency to heal on the surface, leaving underneath large cavities where it becomes rapidly impossible to insert any dressing (Figure 4.4). Small orifices hiding large cavities (Figures 4.5 to 4.7) must be reopened surgically and exposed under their largest surface (Figure 4.8).

UNDERMINING

Some cavities are life threatening, like the trochanteric pressure ulcer when undermining creates an opening of the hip capsule, located close to the basis of the femoral

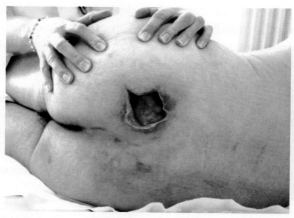

Figure 4.2: Incision of one side of a contracted skin located over a large deep cavity can provide enough access to the wound management

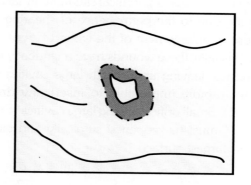

Figure 4.3: Drawing representing the extent of the undermined area

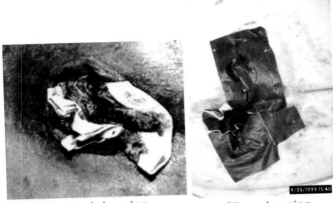

Charcoal dressing   **Silver dressing**

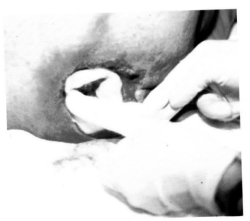

Alginate

Figure 4.4: Cavity wounds can be problematic when located close to an orifice. Negative pressure therapy can be used immediately after sharp debridement

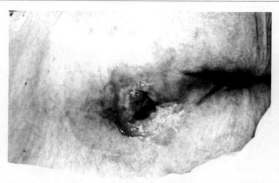

Figure 4.5: After proper treatment, reduction of the wound size by contraction and granulation tissue formation

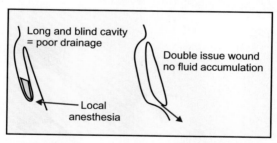

Figure 4.6: Long blind cavities cannot be drained. Under local anesthesia, an efficient drainage can be obtained

neck, and provokes an osteoarthritis of the hip **(Figures 4.9 and 4.10)**. On an unsensible paraplegic patient, this situation progresses towards a complete destruction of the femoral head, and lately, towards a brutal rupture of the femoral artery and vein, susceptible to cause a fatal hemorrhage **(Figure 4.11)**. This complication is observed when shearing forces are applied on the wound, or when

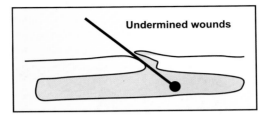

Figure 4.7: Undermined areas can be observed during the post-operative period, in pressure sores and diabetic foot ulcers. The diagnosis can only be assumed when exploring the wound using a penetrating soft-ended instrument. This exploration is an important element to prevent failures of management of the wounds. When these undermined areas are not recognized properly and treated adequately, the infection develops laterally under the skin surface

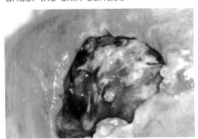

Figure 4.8: Undermining is a real danger. Unknown, it represents one of the main causes of failure reported to a bad choice of the dressing. A correct evaluation of a wound should include exploration of potential undermined areas

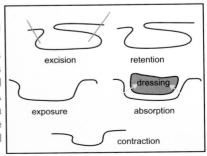

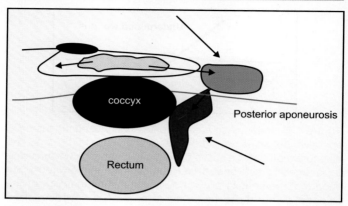

Figure 4.9: Progression of infection from a sacral pressure sore is lateral initially, then across the aponeurosis, laterally to the coccyx, then to the rectum, then in the depth along the lateral aspect of the rectum.

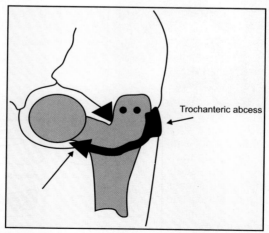

Figure 4.10: Progression of the undermining infection around the femoral neck towards the capsule ends in a hip osteoarthritis imposing head and neck resection

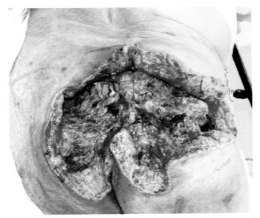

Figure 4.11: Fatal pressure ulcer : sacro-ischio-trochanteric pressure ulcer to debride but septicemia occurs issuing into death

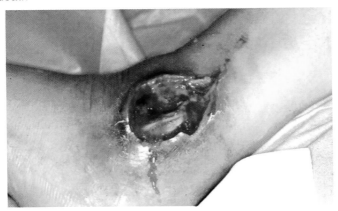

Figure 4.12: Exposure of the tendon imposes immobilization, local anti-infectious agents and a systemic antibiotherapy

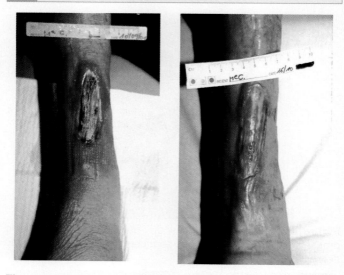

Figure 4.13: When exposed tendon is properly managed, the superficial part of the fibers becomes completely devascularized. Their debridement is possible and must be realized economically. Wound closure can then be obtained, with preservation of a partial tendon (and a partial function)

movements are still allowed when a tendon is exposed **(Figure 4.12)**. In this case, a progressive undermining is seen on the edges of the tendon axposure, which can be long along the tendon, issuing to delay in healing **(Figure 4.13)**.

Chapter 5

Types of Tissues to be Debrided

NECROTIC TISSUE

Mechanical debridement at the bed site can be realized on necrotic tissue (Figure 5.1), fibrous and adherent tissue, undermined areas and local infection (evident or suspected). The necrotic tissue debridement must find the good plan of dissection between necrosis and healthy tissues, which is easy when separation is possible (Figure 5.2), more difficult if adherent (Figure 5.3). "At risks" tissues can be debrided, adjuvant techniques are recommended for tissues at " low risks". A period of 3 to 4 days should be the maximum to obtain a complete debridement.

FIBROTIC TISSUES

Fibrotic tissues are difficult areas to debride (Figure 5.4). Tissues are adherent, and debridement is painful. Bleeding is a frequent adverse event. To help such debridement curette, scissors and repeated aggressive stages are completed usually with moisturizing dressings change everyday (Figure 5.5). Some of fibrotic tissues are intermingled between granulation tissue (e.g. venous leg ulcer), others are repetitively seen on the surface of the wound in case of important devascularization (e.g. arterial leg ulcer). Fibrous tissue can be observed also in cancer wounds, a situation when debridement must not be extensive if painful.

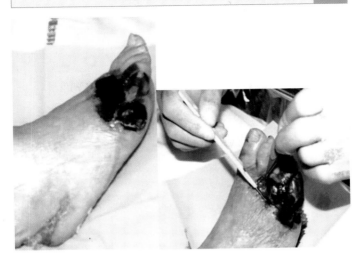

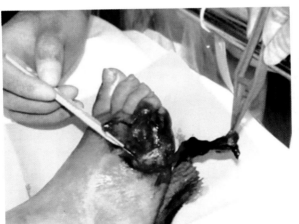

Figure 5.1: In association with revascularization (by pass or angiopalsty), sharp debridement of necrosis is recommended to limit the risk of amputation

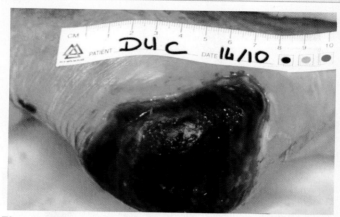

Figure 5.2: Heel pressure ulcer associated with arterial insufficiency with dry eschar need can be debrided if edema, erythema, fluctuance or drainage are present and if revascularization is done before

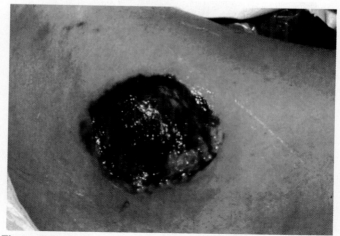

Figure 5.3: To promote healing and to prevent infection a sharp debridement associated with autolytic one with absorbent dressing is required

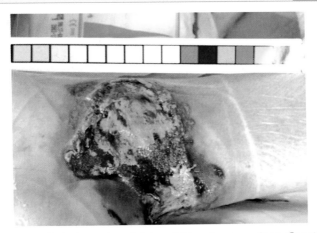

Figure 5.4: Adherent, painful and bleeding leg ulcer. Curette, scissors, repeated aggressive stages should be used. Moisturizing dressings are needed

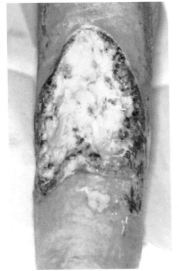

Figure 5.5: Debride yellow sloughy tissue to prevent infection and promote granulation in venous leg ulcer

INFECTED AND SLOUGHY TISSUES

Infected areas should be tretated like necrotic zones, keeping in mind the necessity to increase locally the extent of debridement (Figure 5.6), and repeat the

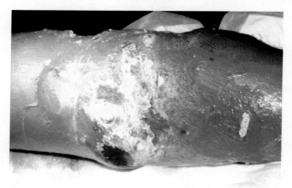

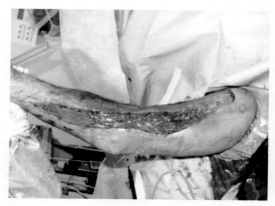

Figure 5.6: Subcutaneous upper limb infection after cocaine injection: Extensive debridement, lavage, granulation, skin grafting

debridement if necessary everyday until complete resection of sloughy materials and cavities. Bleeding is more important when inflammation and infection are more marked.

In infected wound, soft tissue are to be debrided, cavities to be exposed (Figures 5.7 to 5.9), fistulae to be drained and infected bone to be debrided (Figures 5.10 and 5.11). Infected bone should be treated by general antibiotics or limited resection, as negative pressure therapy and flap or graft.

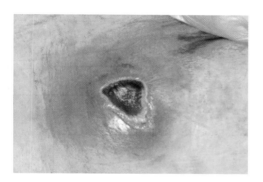

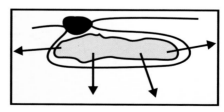

Figure 5.7: Hyperthermia without evident cause can be lately reported to the pressure ulcer covered with a small necrotic cover

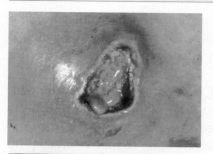

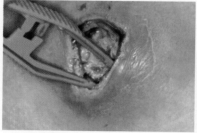

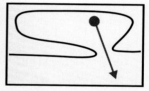

Figure 5.8: Excision without anesthesia of the necrotic cover
at the bedside evacuates pus

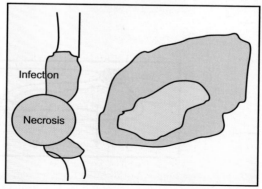

Figure 5.9: Drawing representing, around the necrotic area,
the extent of the infected zone

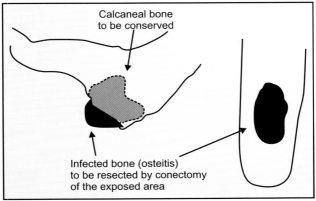

Figure 5.10: Schematic lateral view of the osteitic part of the calcaneus

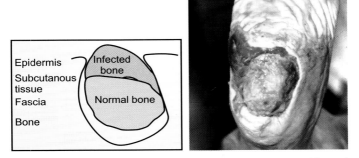

Figure 5.11: Osteitis of the calcaneus is a local problem. Most of the time, "marsupialization" of the protruding infected bone will be sufficient to find the normal bone. On this sole, the granulation tissue will develop and the wound will close

Chapter 6

Types of Etiologies

Debridement can be surgical, autolytic, biological or enzymatic. Which debridement for which situation should be adopted? This is a matter of discussion even in most sophisticated units. A technique of debridement can be choosen just because of the local facilities, the sensibility of the nursing staff, or the disponibility of an operating room not far around. Surgery is always a tendency adopted when possible **(Figure 6.1)**. In specialized clinics (DFU, PU, VLU) most of the debridement is done without any help of surgeons by professionals surrounding the patient. A trained nurse in these clinics knows more than a professor of surgery who never practices. In this chapter, we try to present the most usual techniques adopted

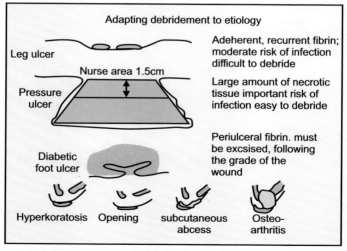

Figure 6.1: Different types of wounds can be observed, into which different types of debridement should be proposed

everywhere in the world to each clinical situation. These proposals should be adapted locally.

PRESSURE SORES

See **Figures 6.2 to 6.7**.

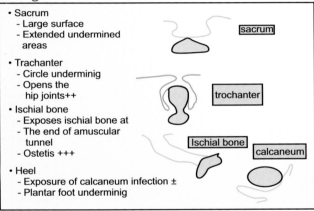

- Sacrum
  - Large surface
  - Extended undermined areas
- Trachanter
  - Circle underminig
  - Opens the hip joints++
- Ischial bone
  - Exposes ischial bone at
  - The end of amuscular tunnel
  - Ostetis +++
- Heel
  - Exposure of calcaneum infection ±
  - Plantar foot underminig

sacrum

trochanter

Ischial bone   calcaneum

Figure 6.2: Different shapes of cavities in pressure ulcers

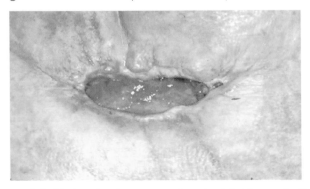

Figure 6.3: Undermined pressure ulcer to debride surgically if total wound closure is expected

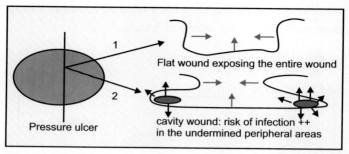

Figure 6.4: Same visual aspect, two different anatomical situations. Visual evaluation is not enough when assessing wounds. Soft ended instruments evaluation is as important as visual one

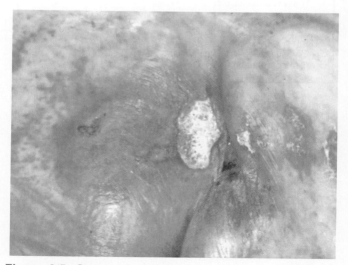

Figure 6.5: Stage 3 sacral pressure ulcer. Not to debride surgically. Autolytic debridement using for example hydrocolloid should be sufficient

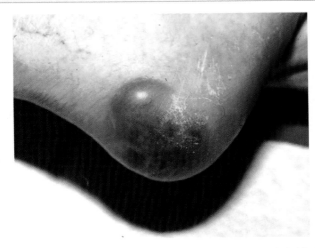

Figure 6.6: Stage 2 pressure ulcer: blister must be debride in order to prevent infection

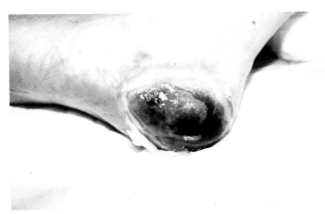

Figure 6.7: Stage 4 heel pressure ulcer. Debridement will be first realized using moist dressing (hydrogel) and afterwards using scalpel and scissors

DIABETIC FOOT ULCER

See **Figures 6.8 to 6.15**.

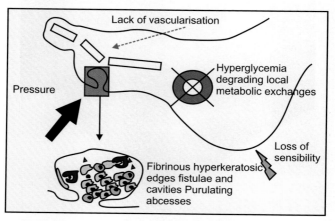

Figure 6.8: Multiple causative factors in diabetic foot ulcer

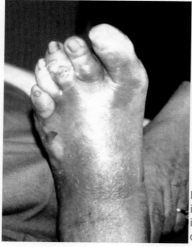

Figure 6.9: If debridement is not sufficient enough, infection occurs very quickly in diabetic foot ulcer

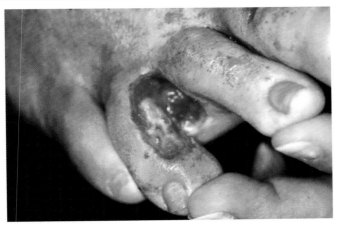

Figure 6.10: Diabetic foot debridement: debridement converts a hidden cavity into an open free of germs cavity

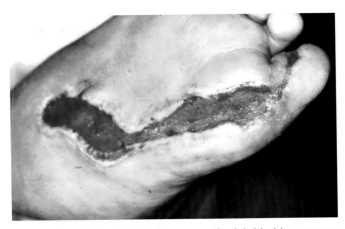

Figure 6.11: Diabetic foot ulcer correctly debrided by surgeon. Moist wound healing using adapted dressing can now be proposed until obtaining total wound closure

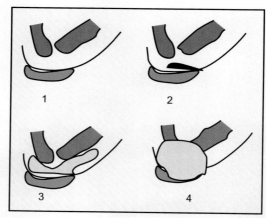

Figure 6.12: (1) Hyperkeratosis, (2) Skin break due to shearing forces between the hyperkeratosic area and the normal skin, (3) Development of undermined cavity, (4) Involvement of the metatarso-phalangeal joint: osteoarthritis

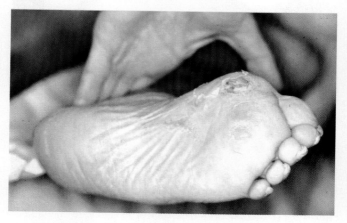

Figure 6.13: Hyperkeratosic area on a diabetic foot

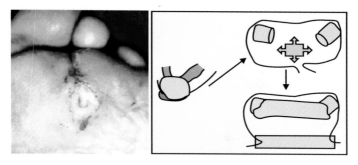

Figure 6.14: Diabetic foot ulcer: debridement converts a hidden cavity into an open free of germs cavity

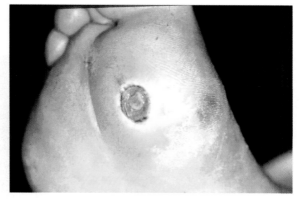

Figure 6.15: Diabetic foot ulcer to be debrided in order to improve wound healing and to prevent infection

AMPUTATION STUMP

See **Figures 6.16 to 6.18**

VENOUS LEG ULCER

See **Figures 6.19 to 6.25**

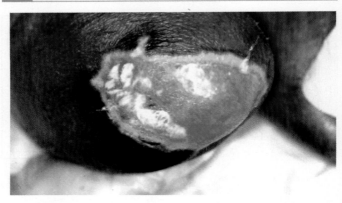

Figure 6.16: Amputation stump in leprotic patient should be smoothly debrided using adapted dressings

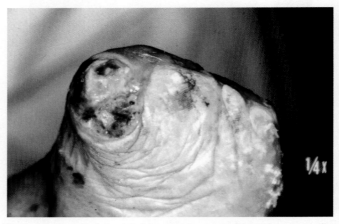

Figure 6.17: Autolytic debridement is needed for this amputation stump. Hydrogel under occlusive dressing like polyurethane film or thin hydrocolloid or foam is recommended

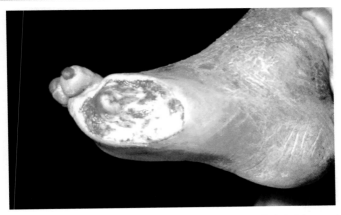

Figure 6.18: In this amputation stump surgical debridement should be associated with flap to prevent bacterial bone recontamination

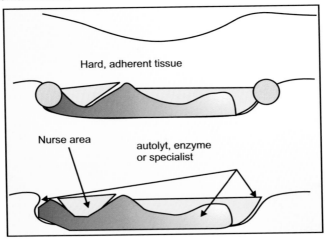

Figure 6.19: Venous leg ulcer is a typical flat wound, whose characteristics are a middle size wound, sloping gently edges typically located on the anterolateral aspect of the distal tibia, provoking a sound pain, presenting a high tendency to exudate

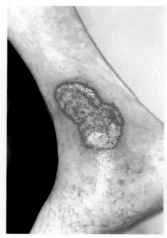

Figure 6.20: Venous leg ulcer to be debrided using for example alginate dressing or using saline on gauze daily changed

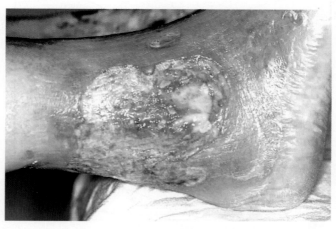

Figure 6.21: After application of EMLA cream, it is necessary to debride yellow dead tissue on the wound bed of this venous leg ulcer using curette

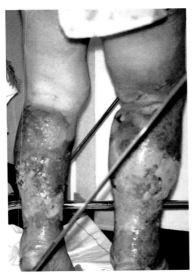

Figure 6.22: A bath with soap prepares this leg to debridement. Local anesthesia is not possible here on such large area, so autolytic debridement with alginate dressing or hydrofiber is required

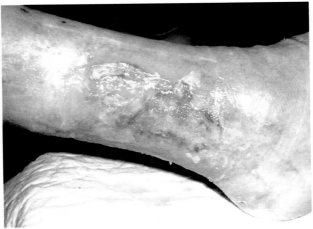

Figure 6.23: It is not absolutely needed to debride a non-infected wound, with few necrotic tissue, foreign matter or fibrin slough

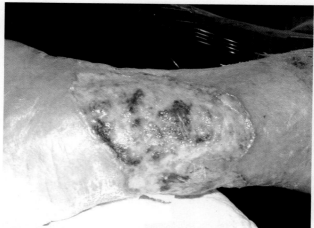

Figure 6.24: To debride leg ulcer, remove with forceps devitalized tissues in the aim here to prevent infection

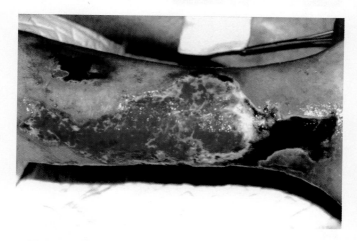

Figure 6.25: Necrotizing fasciitis debrided using autolytic debridement

ARTERIAL LEG ULCER

See **Figures 6.26 to 6.32**.

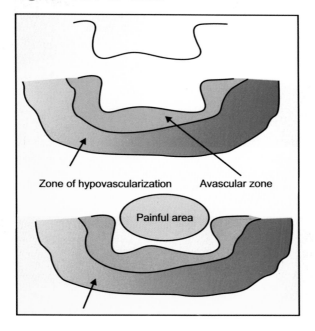

Zone of hypovascularization   Avascular zone

Painful area

Figure 6.26: Arterial leg ulcer is a moderate size wound on the anterior middle aspect of the tibia, sloping sharply edges, extremely painful, without tendency to heal

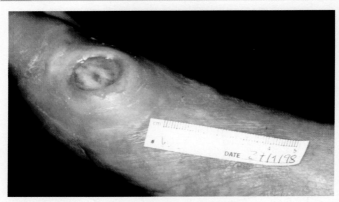

Figure 6.27: In this arterial foot ulcer debridement is needed to prevent infection. Angioplasty or arterial by-pass should also be realized in order to restore local vascularization and to promote wound healing

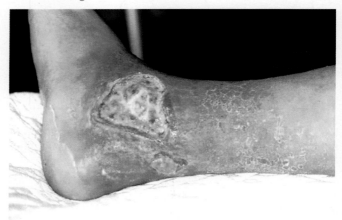

Figure 6.28: Arguments in favot of a mixt origin in a leg ulcer are: same localization than a venous leg ulcer, more deep, less granulation tissue, more painful, longer to heal. Debridement is here required after local anesthesia

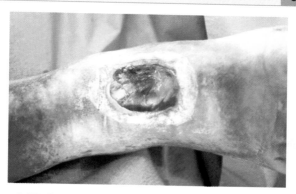

Figure 6.29: On this mixt ulcer, debridement is needed to remove all necrotic tissues. Tendon is visible on the wound bed and will also probably be removed

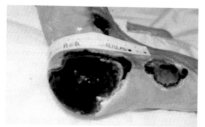

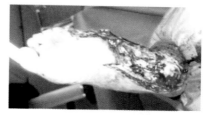

Figure 6.30: In the operating room "carcinologic" excision is needed. Infection control should include exposure of all undermined areas and cavities. Debridement should be associated with revascularization. The moment for amputation has to be defined precisely with the vascular surgeon

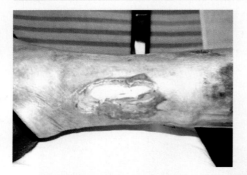

Figure 6.31: When the joints around the wound are immobilized, tendon exposure is limited to the wound area (1), When mobilisation is maintained, a long undermining infected tunnel is often observed on both sides of the tendon exposure (2)

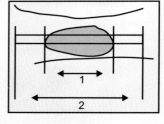

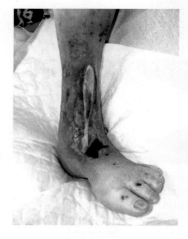

Figure 6.32: This necrotic tendon has to be cut. In arterial insufficiency, debridement is required in this association with revascularization procedure in order to prevent amputation

MALIGNANT WOUNDS

See Figures 6.33 to 6.35.

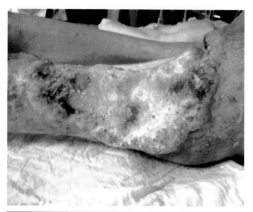

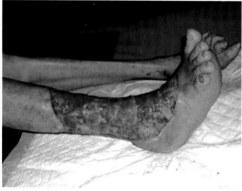

Figure 6.33: A large surgical and "carcinologic" debridement was conducted in this squamous cell carcinoma developed on a chronic leg ulcer with more than 20 years of duration

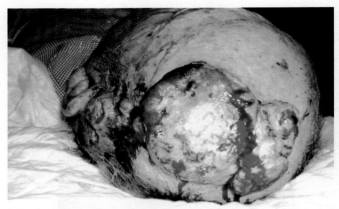

Figure 6.34: Alternative diagnosis should be evoked before debriding a chronic wound: here a squamous cell carcinoma on an amputation stump

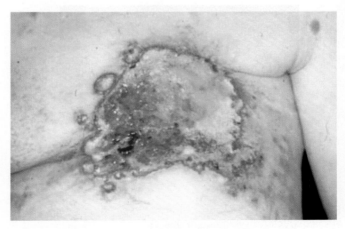

Figure 6.35: Breast cancer. Malignant painful wound. No debridement is needed

BURNS

See **Figures 6.36 and 6.37**.

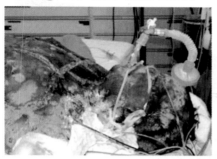

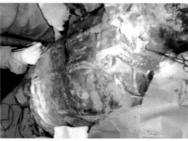

Figure 6.36: In burns debridement has to be adapted to the depth of the burns and the extent of the burnt surface

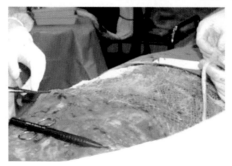

Figure 6.37: In burns after debridement skin grafts are necessary

HEMATOMA

See Figure 6.38.

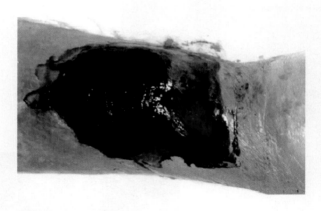

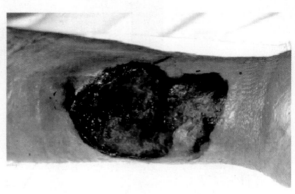

Figure 6.38: Leg hematoma in a patient under anticoagulation can create a large wound highly susceptible of becoming infected. Debridement has to be quickly realized. No pain, no bleeding in the ward is possible, alginates dressing being of resources in these situations

TRAUMATIC DERMABRASIONS

See Figure 6.39.

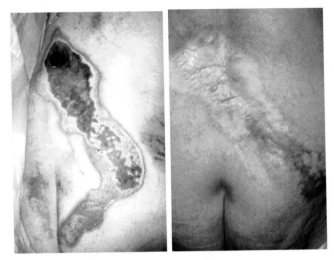

Figure 6.39: Dermabrasion of the back in an old patient with healing, without using mechanical debridement, only autolytic debridement with hydrocolloid dressings

LACERATION

See **Figure 6.40**.

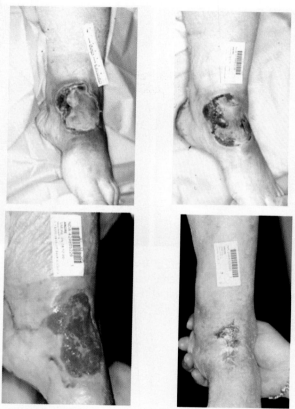

Figure 6.40: Debridement has to be realized in a proper timing. After a surgical procedure having debrided extensively the wound bed, failure of a covering flap does not need an urgent reoperation. After sometimes, a good wound bed will be found when removing the necrosed tissue

SKIN TEARS

See **Figures 6.41 and 6.42**

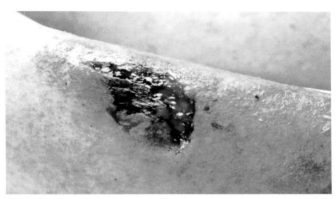

Figure 6.41: Skin tears are often seen after trauma in elderly
population on the anterior aspect of the leg

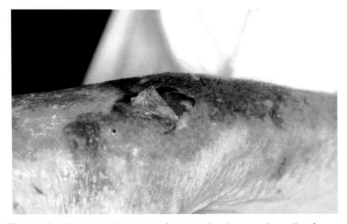

Figure 6.42: Lacerations are frequently observed on the face,
the scalp, the lower limbs of very old patients

SURGICAL WOUNDS

See **Figure 6.43**.

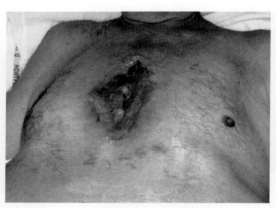

Figure 6.43: Postoperative infection is frequent after sternotomy and coronary bypass; osteitis of the sternal edges are observed. A deep abscess of the anterior mediastinum complicates the capacity to heal. Aspirative drainage (negative pressure therapy is recommended)

PSYCHIATRIC WOUNDS

See **Figures 6.44 and 6.45**

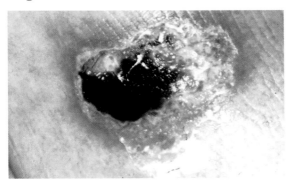

Figure 6.44: Necrotic tissue can be limited and surrounded by a granulation tissue. Debridement should be very selective and limited

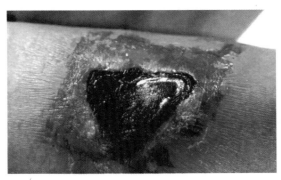

Figure 6.45: Dry black necrosis caused by an external agent in psychiatric patient if after occlusion dressing is possible and specialist management

CONCLUSION

See **Figure 6.46**.

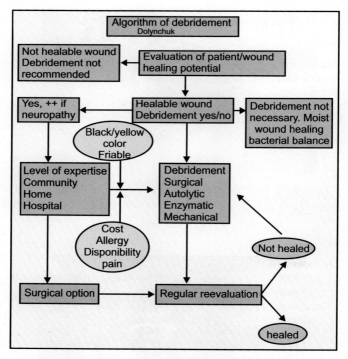

Figure 6.46: Algorithm of debridement (following Dolynchuk)

Index

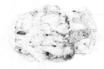